100 Habits of Highly Successful Weight Losers

By Brad Watkins M.D.

Dedicated to

My wife, Pamela
Our beautiful twins, Morgan & Kendall

Our Labrador retriever, Bella

Cover designed by Kendall Watkins

Introduction

Weight loss is hard.

If it were easy, we wouldn't have an obesity epidemic in the United States after 50+ years of diet plans and books. Our bodies are programmed for survival. The ability to store calories is a powerful mechanism for this goal. Generations of people before us strengthened the gene pool as those less resilient to famine died. Our ancestors that excelled at storing calories survived. For survival, our physiological processes defend weight gain. When we try to lose weight, our body puts up a fight. If it thinks for an instant that famine is coming, it sounds the alarm and all systems go to battle station.

The myriad weight loss recommendations contradict and confuse us. Baked potato. Grapefruit. South Beach. Weight Watchers. Zone. Atkins. Paleo. Volumetrics. Keto, etc. An old adage in medicine says, "If there is more than one way to do things, that means none of them work very well." Advice for the best weight loss strategy varies widely.

Consistent myths are pervasive and cause frustration from lack of results. They are worth mentioning:

Myth #1 – *Weight loss is simple.* It is not simple. If it were, we wouldn't have a rising obesity epidemic in the U.S.

Myth #2 – *The same weight loss plan works for everyone.* Weight loss is complex. Humans are complex. The solution to obesity is complex.

Myth #3 – *If I do nutrition perfect, I will lose weight.* Mental stuff and fitness are equally important disciplines to master for sustainable long-term success.

Myth #4 – *You can lose weight without changing your eating and fitness habits.* Successful weight losers make many significant changes. Your ability to change determines your success to achieve and maintain a healthy weight.

Myth #5 – *Someday we will have a magic pill that will make me lose weight without changing any of my habits.* We will never have this pill. We can stop looking for it.

Why should we even care about obesity? Obesity increases the risk of many medical conditions such as dying at a younger age, cancer, heart attack, stroke, diabetes, high blood pressure, high cholesterol, joint pain, sleep apnea and infertility, just to name a few. Obesity is now the #1 cause of preventable death in the United States. This used to be smoking, but the obesity epidemic now kills more people than cigarettes. The good news is that most obesity-related health problems are reversible with successful weight loss. I experienced this with my own health. My first year out of residency, I finally had time to eat and 24-hour access to a fully stocked doctor's lounge at the hospital. I quickly gained 30 pounds and ended up on medications for high blood pressure and cholesterol. It took me months of avoiding the doctor's lounge and a lot of hard work to get back to a healthy weight and stop taking medications. My weight has been a daily battle since.

After working in a weight loss clinic for nearly 20 years, I've had many patients lose a lot of weight and others that didn't lose very much. Whenever we study our top 25% of weight losers and compare them to the bottom 25%, consistent characteristics emerge. When a patient loses over 100 lbs, their friends and co-workers always ask the same question: "What are you doing?" Asking someone who has successfully completed a difficult task is smart.

There are countless weight loss books published by experts but the real experts are the patients who have just lost over 100 pounds. People don't tend to finish thick heavy books that are hard to understand. This weight loss book is thin and easy to read. If you want to know how to climb Mount Everest, ask people who have signed the logbook in the thin air atop the summit. They are the true experts. There are many theories and detailed explanations of the endocrine system, but what works? I work in a busy weight loss clinic with some of the best professionals in the business. I am a surgeon but this is not a surgical book. All weight loss patients (surgical and medical) have to make the same changes and healthy decisions for success. Over many years, our successful weight losers have taught us valuable lessons for anyone on this journey. The highly successful weight losers have distinctive habits in common. Do you want to know how to lose weight? Ask the experts. Do you want to know what the experts have done? Read on.

Weight Loss 101

I'm not sure we understand everything we know about this.

Anonymous

Three legged stool

The three disciplines of successful weight loss are the mental stuff, fitness and nutrition. Think of them like a three-legged stool. If you take one away, the whole thing falls down. I see many patients who have perfect nutrition logs and they wonder why they're not losing weight, but their calorie burning is zero so they remain in positive calorie balance not to mention a lower metabolism from inactivity. If these patients simply add a walking regimen to their daily schedule, they will start losing weight. Similarly, I have female patients with a history of sexual abuse and though their nutrition and fitness are perfect, without addressing the mental stuff, they will sabotage when men pay closer attention to them.

Far too often, people try to nutrition their way to weight loss with no calorie burning. Or they try to gym their way to weight loss with no regard to nutrition. And none of this works without addressing the mental stuff. I purposefully put this section at the front of this book to emphasize the importance of the mental stuff. Successful weight losers have a well thought out plan for all three. They work hard and get results and maintain a healthy weight.

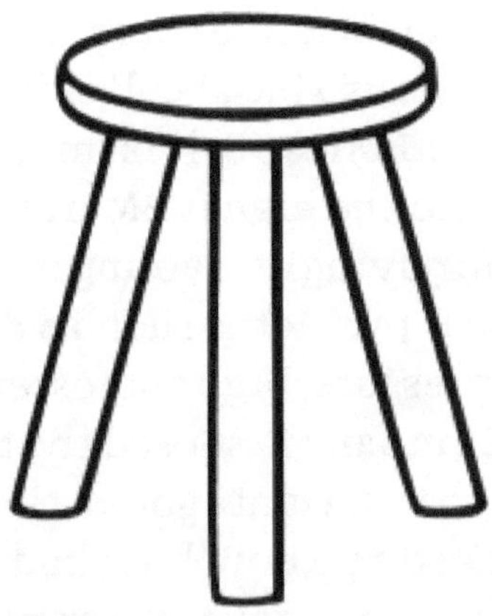

Go back in time

In the 1970s, obesity rates in the U.S. were low and stable. We were more active and we ate fewer calories. We weren't eating fried potatoes three times per day in our car. Dessert was reasonable and occasional. We didn't have brilliant food chemistry like high fructose corn syrup and trans fats. We ate at the dining room table with our families – not in our car, in front of the TV or computer or at our desks. We have so radically distorted the norms of eating and activity level, the mere suggestion of not eating fried potatoes three times per day in your car make people look at you like you are crazy. Dr. David Kessler, former FDA commissioner says we need "food rehab". We have radically distorted norms. We have to go back in time. We have to re-establish these societal norms.

Know your BMI

BMI = Body Mass Index. BMI takes your height and weight into account so it is a better indicator of how unhealthy you are than simply looking at your weight in pounds.

BMI 25 – 30   Overweight
BMI 30 – 35   Class I Obesity
BMI 35 – 40   Class II Obesity (Severe Obesity)
BMI 40 – 50   Class III Obesity (Morbid Obesity)
BMI > 50   Super Obesity

From a health perspective, there is a big difference between a

BMI of 30 and a BMI of 60 just like there is a big difference between the health implications of a basal cell skin cancer and metastatic ovarian cancer. If your BMI is 30, it is important to lose weight to prevent escalating into the higher BMI ranges. If your BMI is >40, you are higher risk for dying at a younger age, higher risk for cancer and many medical problems such as diabetes, heart attacks, strokes, high blood pressure, high cholesterol, etc. The Metropolitan Life Insurance Company first used the term "Morbid Obesity" because they knew that patients above this BMI didn't live a normal life span. You need to know how bad your disease is so that you understand the need to make an aggressive plan if your BMI is greater than 40.

Get your labs checked

A common reason to give up on a weight loss attempt is frustration with poor results. Sometimes poor results are due to an undiagnosed medical condition. It is important to get a physical from your doctor and have them check several important labs. In addition to the normal battery of labs, here is a list of important labs for your doctor to order:

> Vitamin D
> Thyroid panel
> Cortisol
> Testosterone

Medical conditions that can work hard against your weight loss efforts include low Vitamin D, hypothyroid (low thyroid), elevated cortisol (Cushing's Disease) and low testosterone. Testosterone is associated with muscle mass, which is the biggest contributor to our metabolism (BMR- basal metabolic rate). Low testosterone in men will lower their metabolism and make it very difficult to lose weight. Female testosterone levels are much lower than males but if lower than normal, this can cause depression, low sex drive and weight gain. Replacing testosterone to normal levels can improve weight loss success in men and women.

Stop or change medications associated with weight gain

Some medications cause us to gain weight. They can increase our appetite, slow our metabolism, or encourage our bodies to store calories. Frequently, your doctor can change your medications to alternatives that treat the same condition without weight gain. Steroids can cause weight gain. Some medications that treat high blood pressure, seizures, anxiety, depression and diabetes can cause weight gain. Talk to your doctor.

It is also important to realize that as you lose weight, your blood pressure and diabetes will improve. If you don't adjust your medications accordingly, your blood pressure and/or blood sugar may get too low. This can cause syncopal episodes (faint, pass out) that cause injury. It is very important to monitor your blood pressure and blood sugar closely as you lose weight or you could faint and injure yourself.

General health

Similar to getting a physical before you play sports in high school, it is important to get a physical before you lose weight. This can identify undiagnosed problems. For example, some patients don't realize they are pre-diabetic, etc. Your doctor needs to have a game plan to monitor medications as you lose weight. Depending on your age they might also recommend testing such as electrocardiogram (EKG), mammogram, colonoscopy, etc. as a routine part of health screening exams.

Recognize that 2 lbs per week is a healthy weight loss

Everyone wants to lose 100 pounds overnight and get discouraged when this doesn't happen, but a healthy, natural weight loss is 1-2 pounds per week. This is a fat-burning weight loss with no muscle wasting.

Lose fat, not muscle

For healthy weight loss, you want to lose stored energy (fat), not muscle. Losing muscle mass will lower your metabolism which makes weight loss harder and is unhealthy. Aggressive diets that make the scale look better by losing muscle are not healthy and not recommended. Patients with malabsorption (reduced nutrient absorption in the GI tract) can lose weight from muscle wasting but this is not healthy.

Websites

Many excellent websites help with weight loss. These include calorie trackers, healthy recipes and guidelines. Most restaurants list nutrition facts on their websites. Here's a list of websites you may find helpful on your journey.

www.FitDay.com
www.CalorieKing.com
www.AllRecipes.com
www.CookingLight.com/magazine
www.myplate.gov
www.nutritiondata.self.com
www.health.gov/dietaryguidelines
www.nutritionfacts.org

Mental stuff

There are no secrets to success. Don't waste time looking for them. Success is the result of perfection, hard work, learning from failure, loyalty to those for whom you work and persistence.

Colin Powell

You are not alone

Many patients are too hard on themselves and get into a mental state that is not helpful. Patients will say they cannot believe they let themselves get this way. It is important to realize that you are not alone. Obesity affects a large percentage of the population. You have to be kind to yourself and understand positive self-talk for successful weight loss. Weight loss attempts in a supportive environment are more successful than going it alone.

Fail

Wait, did you say FAIL? Yes I did. But, this is a book about successful weight loss. Yes it is. A far too common scenario is a patient succeeding at weight loss, but then they eat a candy bar one day and the wheels come completely off the cart. They toss the whole plan out the window and the weight comes back on and brings friends with it. It is important to know that no human is perfect every day. A person who fails is a person who is trying to succeed. Wayne Gretzky said, "You miss 100% of the shots you don't take." All or none thinking will not help your weight loss success. Do not plan for failure, but if you have a bad moment, get back in the saddle and keep working hard.

A TV news station fired a young news anchor. Her name is Oprah Winfrey. A high school basketball team cut one of its players. His name is Michael Jordan. Two Japanese engineers invented a rice cooker that failed because it burned the rice. Their company is Sony. Successful people use failure as a launching pad for success. If you have a bad day, use it to launch you into the stratosphere of success. Imagine a world where Oprah, Michael Jordan and the Sony engineers simply quit and walked away.

The cornerstones of <u>success</u> are honesty, responsibility, commitment and inner strength.

The cornerstones of <u>failure</u> are excuses, blaming, cutting corners, procrastination, giving up easily, enabling saboteurs, dwelling in the past and immediate gratification.

Now, go get back on the horse!

Read *Shrink Yourself* by Roger Gould MD

Dr. Gould is a UCLA psychiatrist who has worked with weight loss patients for many years. His powerful book details patterns of negative psychological energy that we treat with food. He explains the importance of getting to the root of this negative psychological energy for successful weight loss. One of my favorite examples in the book is a patient whose career goal was to get paid to sing. But a boyfriend in high school made fun of her singing and she took a different path. She struggled to lose weight. Once Dr. Gould identified this, he encouraged her to get a job singing. She did and the weight started coming off.

This book has helped many of my patients and deepened my understanding of the mental aspects of weight loss success. I think you will find it valuable.

Change

Expecting weight loss results without making changes is not realistic. Successful weight losers make many changes. Expect to make changes. Humans hate change but successful behavior change is a key aspect of successful weight loss. Some patients have intense past experiences that drive behaviors contributing to weight gain. They may need professional CBT (cognitive behavior therapy) from a specialist to overcome these obstacles and succeed at weight loss. Thoughts and attitudes influence behavior. CBT seeks to explore, surface and understand past experiences that drive compensatory behavior. For example, if you treat pain from a nasty divorce with food, this can require hard work with a professional to cure this association with unhealthy behavior.

Be happy

Untreated depression is a common reason people struggle with weight loss. There are multiple depression screening tools online (Google, "depression screening"). Take a depression-screening test online or talk to your doctor.

Feeling lousy can interrupt the noblest attempt at weight loss. Many times, the lousy feeling is preventable. I see patients who sugar crash from overeating sweets and carbs or poorly managed diabetes medications. Low blood sugar makes them feel lousy so they eat sugar to feel better and they don't lose weight. Losing weight improves blood pressure. I see patients who don't monitor their blood pressure during successful weight loss and adjust their blood pressure medications accordingly. They feel lousy because their blood pressure is too low and they flip right back into bad habits to feel better and they don't lose weight. It is important not to feel lousy when trying to lose weight.

Be miserable

Wait, did you just tell us to be miserable? Yes I did. But you just told us to be happy. Correct. The point here is not to be happy with your disease. If your BMI is over 30, you are at higher risk for many medical diseases that will shorten your life and lower the quality of the life you have left. Successful weight losers are miserable being obese and highly motivated to achieve a healthy weight. I saw an obese patient interviewed on a talk show one day and she told the audience she was "fat and happy" and that her loved ones should just accept that. The audience cheered. This horrified me. We should not celebrate a disease that is the #1 cause of preventable death in the United States. If a friend tells you they have diabetes, cheering would not be an appropriate reaction. If you are not miserable being obese, it will be more difficult to lose weight.

You may need professional help

One thing that shocks and saddens me is the number of obese patients with a history of sexual abuse. Here's a scenario: A young woman was sexually abused as a child. Food becomes a readily available and highly successful treatment for deep emotional trauma. The resulting obesity is a shield of armor because it reduces male attention. Men pay closer attention to her as she loses weight so she sabotages to get her shield of armor back. If this is you, don't attempt to go it alone. Get help. Weight loss success probably requires help from a psychology professional with expertise in this field. This is also true of patients with a history of bulimia or anorexia. If you have a heart issue, don't hesitate to see a cardiologist. If you have a psychological issue, don't hesitate to see a psychology professional.

Intrinsic focus of control

Successful weight loss requires what psychologists call an intrinsic focus of control. I see many obese patients with an extrinsic focus of control.

Example of <u>intrinsic focus of control</u>: *I am in control of my destiny. I control my future and can affect my personal outcome by my actions. I will work hard and persevere to improve my life.*

Example of <u>extrinsic focus of control</u>: *My job caused my knee pain that prevents me from exercising so that is why I can't lose weight. My weight was normal until I had my son so it is his fault that I gained 200 pounds. My obesity is the government's fault because they didn't put warning labels on foods with unhealthy additives. I'm too busy to lose weight because I have four kids and a lazy husband and I have to work. I can't lose weight because it will make my girlfriend jealous and my husband is mean and I have to eat to control my dizziness and the mall closes too early for me to walk and our neighborhood doesn't have sidewalks and my cousin's dog just had puppies and the moon phase is not perfect and I'm waiting for my husband to fix the leaky faucet and...*

Successful weight loss requires an intrinsic focus of control.

Celebrate without food

Your co-worker just treated you to a huge dinner to celebrate your promotion. Your husband just got the top sales award so you celebrate at your favorite Italian restaurant. You get ice cream after every one of your son's baseball games. You go to dinner every time your college roommate comes to town and also your sorority sisters, cousins, aunts, uncles, grandparents, in-laws, and the list goes on and on and on and on. Your husband takes you to dinner for your birthday, Valentines Day, Sweetest Day, Thanksgiving, Christmas, New Years, anniversary, Mother's Day, your kids' birthdays, Labor Day, Memorial Day, President's Day, Columbus Day...

We use food to celebrate. The problem is we have too many celebrations and they are typically high calorie events. Successful weight losers find new ways to celebrate without consuming over 1,000 calories at one sitting.

Accountability

You will be more successful if you weigh-in regularly and report your progress to someone whom you deeply care for. This can be a spouse, a friend, a family member or a weight loss professional. Do you value the opinion of anyone in your life? Report your weight loss to that person. You will be more motivated to lose weight and ultimately more successful.

Support

Weight loss makes a terrible solo sport. One of the biggest predictors of long-term weight loss is support. People trying to lose weight alone are generally not as successful. Weight loss is hard and you need someone to cheer you on and keep you motivated during the tough times.

Phantom hunger

Successful weight losers have a solid understanding of phantom hunger. We teach ourselves to be hungry all the time. If you eat in front of your TV, then you will be hungry every time you turn on the TV because your brain anticipates the pattern that food is coming. If you eat in front of your computer, then you will be hungry every time you turn on your computer. If you eat drive-thru meals in your car, then every time you get in your car, you will be hungry. True hunger is a result of not eating for 4 hours. Patients frequently tell me they are hungry all the time. This is not normal physiologic hunger. This is phantom hunger. You don't see obese animals in the wild. They don't do this. If newborn babies are not hungry, they have no interest in milk. They eat when they have true hunger. When they don't have true hunger, they don't eat. If we only ate when we had true physiological hunger we'd all be thin. We train ourselves like dogs to be "hungry" all the time and ravenous hunger is the most common disruptor to serious weight loss attempts.

True physiologic hunger comes when it's been four hours since you ate and your blood sugar is low and your tummy is rumbling. True hunger is patient. It can wait and any food will do. There is no associated guilt when eating in response to true hunger. This normal physiological reaction occurs about three times per day.

Phantom hunger or mental hunger is a response to a feeling or emotion (I'm bored. He was mean to me). Phantom hunger is panicky (If I don't eat NOW someone will get hurt). Phantom hunger craves specific foods (If I don't get some chocolate right now the universe as we know it will end). If you feel guilty after eating, you probably were eating due to phantom hunger.

Distraction is an important principle to fight phantom hunger. Quite simply, distract yourself with something else. Get a new hobby. Learn to knit. Learn Spanish. Assemble a model car or airplane. Build a dollhouse. Find something else to do to take your mind off the old unhealthy habit. Stop eating in the car or in front of the computer or TV. Successful weight losers develop new sustainable habits.

We develop many abnormal relationships with food that are harmful to our health. We eat to celebrate. We eat to mourn. We eat when we're bored, happy, sad or lonely. Our celebrations and traditions are deeply embedded with food. Eating simply to sustain life has become nearly secondary in our culture.

Most of us are guilty of emotional eating. If emotional eating is destructive to healthy weight loss you have to RIP it (Recognize you have a problem, Identify triggers, Plan of action). Recognize you have a problem – don't deny it. Identify your triggers – list them on a sheet of paper. Make a plan to fight emotional eating. Examples would include recognizing that you eat when you're bored so you need to find things to do such as go for walks, spend time with friends or get a new hobby. If you find that you eat when someone makes you upset you must identify this and make the person aware when and why they made you upset. This conflict must be fixed for the phantom hunger to go away. Food is a great comforter. Successful weight losers find other ways to comfort themselves in order to achieve a healthy weight.

Let go of pent-up emotions. Ask yourself: Who are you angry with? What happened in the past that you are still angry about? Was there an embarrassing incident that you still hold inside? Who are you jealous of? Did someone say something hurtful to you that you still feel bad about? Did someone abandon you? Parent? Boyfriend? Divorce? Are you harboring anger with your current spouse or significant other? Consider these options: forgive the other person, confront the person, write a letter, talk to a counselor or pastor and stop abusive relationships.

Along the same line, it is also important to manage stress. No one can eliminate all stress from their life. We all have it. We just have to manage it. Stress makes it hard to lose weight because it puts our bodies in preservation mode. When we're stressed, our bodies want to cling to stored calories so we can fight a tiger. People who manage stress well are far more successful at losing weight. Organization is an important tool to reduce stress.

Sometimes, emotional eating comes from deeply rooted psychological pain and this may require help from a professional. This is true if you have an eating disorder such as bulimia or anorexia or have a history of sexual abuse. Your primary care physician can refer you to a specialist. You can also find professionals on the American Psychological Association website, www.APA.org/helpcenter. Click "Find a Psychologist" on the left of your screen and enter your zip code. You can select providers that specialize in eating disorders or sexual abuse.

Only eat at the dining table

This closely relates to phantom hunger. We eat in our cars or in front of the TV or computer. We train ourselves to be hungry all the time. Successful weight losers only eat at the dining table at mealtime so their cars and computers don't make them hungry all day.

Sleep

If you're not getting enough rest it will be difficult to lose weight. Lack of quality sleep makes you feel lousy and its hard to lose weight when you feel lousy. A common reason for obese people not sleeping well is sleep apnea. The medical term *apnea* describes a period of time with no breathing. Sleep apnea occurs when you stop breathing during periods of deep sleep. When you're overweight the tissue around your airway is overweight. As long as you are awake, your laryngeal muscles keep your airway open. When you go into deep sleep (REM-rapid eye movement, Stage IV sleep) your laryngeal muscles relax and your airway collapses and you stop breathing.

This is one of the vicious cycles of obesity. You gain weight. The tissue around your airway increases. You develop sleep apnea. Your airway collapses. This interrupts quality sleep. You are too tired to exercise. You gain more weight.

You have sleep apnea if anyone has ever told you that you stop breathing when you sleep and then, after a loud snoring sound you start breathing again. Sleep apnea is also more common in obese diabetic men, BMI>45 and neck circumference >17 inches (43cm). You can measure your neck circumference with a measuring tape used for sewing. Also, dress shirt sizes for men have neck circumference in the first number. For example, if your shirt size is 17/33 or higher, you may have sleep apnea. The best way to determine if you have sleep apnea is to have an overnight screening test done in a sleep lab. The most common treatment for sleep apnea is a CPAP machine (continuous positive airway pressure), which will help prevent airway collapse while you sleep.

Sleep apnea is hard on your heart and lungs. It causes right heart strain and pulmonary hypertension. Many obese patients have undiagnosed, untreated severe sleep apnea. Giving obese patients with untreated sleep apnea an opioid prescription is dangerous. When they go home and take a pain pill, they can die in their sleep. Opioids lengthen periods of stage IV (deep) sleep and can lengthen episodes of apnea (no breathing). There are obese patients with untreated sleep apnea leaving outpatient surgery centers every day with a prescription for opioid pain medication. This is very dangerous.

The poor quality of rest associated with untreated sleep apnea can cause daytime sleepiness. Airline pilots and commercial truck drivers are required to have sleep apnea screening as part of their mandatory physicals. You don't want pilots and truck drivers to fall asleep at the wheel. It is scary how common this is among people driving on our interstates.

If you try to lose weight with untreated sleep apnea you will feel lousy and it will make weight loss more difficult. Treating sleep apnea with a CPAP machine will improve the quality of your sleep and help you lose weight. Curing your sleep apnea with successful weight loss is even better.

Baby steps

Here's a common New Year's resolution: *Starting January 1, I am going to eat healthy every day and go to the gym every night.* Within 24 hours, we're off plan, toss the whole thing in the trash and go back to original habits with renewed enthusiasm against pledges to improve health. Every January 1st, a resolution maker occupies every treadmill in the gym. By January 15th, the treadmills are empty. Successful weight losers take baby steps and get back on course quickly after any interruption. Setting realistic sustainable goals are far more productive in the end than ones that quickly end with injury, frustration and no results.

Most of us eat way too much. We only need about 1,200 calories per day (1,400 in men) to sustain life. If you are currently consuming over 2,000 calories per day or more, it is hard to make the abrupt transition to sustenance only calories in one day. Successful weight losers map out baby steps and work down to reasonable caloric consumption. This is more realistic, sustainable and ultimately successful.

Same goes for fitness. If your goal is to jump from sedentary to 10,000 steps per day on the sweet pedometer you just purchased, you probably will get very frustrated or injured and quit. Best to shoot for 1,000 steps per day and then keep moving up your goal until you achieve 10,000 steps per day. The most successful weight losers will get their 10,000 steps in per day but they don't get there in one day.

Motivations

I want to lose weight so I that can date, get married, and have kids. I want to lose weight to get rid of my diabetes. I want to lose weight so I can be more active with my kids. I want to lose weight because I have an autistic child and no one will take care of him like me so I need to live a long healthy life so that I can be around to take care of him. I watched my obese mother die from heart failure and I don't want to die like that.

These are powerful motivators. These are things that some of my most successful weight losers have told me. I've had patients that didn't lose very much weight tell me they are happy in their skin and their spouse loves them and they don't care about losing weight. This is a dangerous attitude.

Find your powerful motivators to lose weight. Write them on an index card. Tape the card to the mirror where you brush your teeth every morning. It will help you lose weight.

Believe in yourself

If you tell yourself you are a failure and you will never lose weight, this is likely to come true. Successful weight losers are kind to themselves and have a positive attitude.

Have you ever wondered why the elephant chained to a tiny

wooden stake doesn't just flick it out of the ground and run free? When the elephant is a baby, they chain its leg to a concrete post and it pulls and tugs for days until it concludes that escape is not possible. It will then spend the rest of its life standing there with a chain around its leg because it *believes* escape is futile.

We used to believe that no human could run a 4-minute mile. Many people tried unsuccessfully. We finally concluded that this feat was not possible for humans to achieve. But on May 6, 1954, Roger Bannister (a physician), ran the mile at Oxford University's Iffley Road Track in 3 minutes and 59.4 seconds. What's even more remarkable about this is how many men ran a sub 4-minute mile in the years following Bannister's incredible achievement. They were successful because they *believed* it was possible.

In a study published in the *Journal of Psychology* in 1972, researchers measured individual arm strength in men before an arm wrestling contest. At each pairing they told the stronger man he was weaker and the weaker man he was stronger and 83% of the time the weaker man won because he *believed* he was stronger. You must know weight loss is possible.

Successful weight losers also have good self-esteem. Low self-esteem fights hard against successful long-term weight loss. Consider taking a daily B-complex vitamin as they help with self-esteem, energy levels and depression.

Be kind to yourself. You can't be your own worst enemy and expect success. If you keep telling yourself you are fat, lazy, and stupid, you will start to believe this after a while. You must be kind to yourself. List things you do well. List accomplishments, graduations, things other people like about you and list things you like about yourself. If you have trouble, ask your mother and she'll come up with pages of material. Have your mother write down your positive attributes on an index card and tape it to the mirror where you brush your teeth every morning.

Reward yourself

Plan the reward you will give yourself when you achieve your goals. Think big. Write it down and tape it to the mirror where you brush your teeth. Tape it beside your list of motivations. Oh, and your reward cannot involve food.

Lose the panicky sense for food

Many people panic about food. Out of fear of being trapped with nothing to eat, we take loads of junk food in the car on long trips. We get obsessed about food. Successful weight losers find healthy obsessions such as tracking calories, healthy cooking and fun ways to burn calories.

Make gradual but lasting changes

Patient #1 – *On January 1, I'm going to run a marathon every day and eat nothing but broccoli.*

Patient #2 – *Starting today, I'm going to get at least 1,000 steps on my pedometer and work up to 10,000 steps per day by the end of the month. I will increase the number of steps each week until I reach my goal. My tracking shows that I am eating over 3,000 calories per day and I seem to prefer higher fat foods. I will reduce my fat gram intake and total calories over time until I reach my goal. If I have a bad day, I will get back on schedule as quickly as possible.*

Which of these two patients do you think will be more successful? You are correct.

Get your mind off hunger

This is incredibly easy to say and hard to do. Many obese patients tell me they are hungry all the time. You have to identify sources of phantom hunger and manage them with a well thought out plan. You have to get your mind on something else when you feel hungry at non-mealtimes. Examples: *I felt hungry so I drank a glass of water and went for a walk. Knitting gets my mind off hunger so when I feel hungry I knit.*

Avoid grazing

Grazing is the term used for cows eating grass all day. When you eat small amounts of food throughout the day instead of at mealtimes you are eating like a cow. Grazing can trickle in large numbers of calories over the course of a day. Successful weight losers don't do this. If you have bowls of snacks positioned around the house or work, you have to get rid of them. If you want to stop smoking you gotta get the cigarettes out of the house.

Self-control is better than willpower

<u>Willpower</u> = *I will not eat the ice cream sitting in the freezer.*
<u>Self-control</u> = *I will not buy ice cream because if it's in the freezer I will eat it.*

Which do you think is more successful? You are correct. Self-control.

Successful weight losers avoid situations where lack of self-control requires massive willpower.

Make yourself a priority

Many patients tell me they have taken care of others for years and now it's time to take care of themselves. They will care for family, aging parents, foster children and others at the expense of their own health. Another option is to prioritize your health so that you can be your best for the people whom you care about the most.

Find sustainable solutions

Many patients try to race from a completely sedentary lifestyle to an intense daily gym routine. Then they get hurt and the whole program is over. This also kills any motivation to start a calorie-burning program in the future. Successful weight losers make rational goals and find sustainable solutions to achieve them.

Set realistic goals

My goal is to lose weight – too generic.

My goal is not to eat ice cream when my husband is out of town – much better, more specific.

Your goals should be specific about the changes you plan to make. I want to lose weight this year - too generic and won't work. I want to increase my walking every week until I reach 10,000 steps per day. Goals should have a measurable quantity so you can monitor your progress. Realistic goals are important to establish momentum and keep it going. Unachievable goals lead to disappointment and failure. Start small and work up.

Recognize sabotage

Sadly, a common human trait is that we don't want other people to be more successful than us. We don't tend to socialize with people who make more money than us. We quietly don't root for friends and family that achieve great success. We tend to hire new employees that won't outshine us instead of hiring the best candidate to move the company in a stronger direction. Many husbands don't want their wives to lose weight because they are afraid they will leave them for another man. I have patients who lost a lot of weight and then their obese friends disown them. Many medical students have people try very hard to talk them out of applying to medical school because this was not an achievable goal for them. Recognize when friends, co-workers or family members selfishly try to sabotage you because they fear your success.

Recruit your team

Weight loss is a team sport. It makes a terrible solo sport. Support is a common element among successful weight losers. They assemble a team of positive people who hold them accountable, pick them up when they fall and cheer them on in moments of victory.

Create competition

Competition is healthy. Companies make better products at a lower price in a competitive market. Humans are innately competitive. What do you do when someone passes you on the freeway? Do you speed up? Use instinctive competitiveness to achieve your weight loss goals. Whenever an office group creates a weight loss competition, you see people that have struggled with diets in the past drop weight consistently with a crazy look in their eye. Get a group of friends, family or co-workers together and create a weight loss competition. Now release your inner Tiger and go kick some @#$%&!

Volunteer

It is hard to lose weight when you feel lousy. The list of items that make you feel lousy is long. It is important to identify and address those items to achieve successful weight loss. One of the most powerful things to make you feel good about yourself is to volunteer. You can find endless opportunities by contacting your local church, school or hospital. Google "volunteer opportunities" and see what comes up. A couple of websites devoted to volunteer opportunities in your area include: www.volunteermatch.org and www.justserve.org

Mindful eating exercise

Medical training taught me how to devour food like a wild animal that hasn't eaten in a week. My wife hates it. This is neither a healthy way to eat nor a successful weight loss method. Try this mindful eating exercise: Arrange on a plate a cashew, a raisin, a slice of apple and a slice of banana. Sit in a dark room. Play meditation music from a "spa" playlist. With slow movements, take one item at a time and let it sit in your mouth and count slowly to 20 (One Mississippi, two Mississippi, etc). Then chew it for a count to 20. Then swallow it. Do the same with each item. As the food item sits in your mouth, concentrate on the complexity of flavors and consistency of each item. Do the same as you chew. Mindful eating can slow you down and get full on a smaller volume of food. This gives more time for the delayed fullness signal to catch up as well.

Meet friends for a walk, not calories

A very popular thing in our culture is to meet friends for lunch or dinner. This typically involves high calorie highly processed restaurant foods. This can make weight loss challenging. Alternatively, you can meet a friend for a walk or a bike ride. Successful weight losers tend to substitute high caloric intake social encounters for ones that burn lots of calories.

Quit your job

Why would you tell me to quit my job? I have patients who lose weight after quitting a stressful job. Others gain a lot of weight after a promotion to a managerial desk job. I also have many patients who went from a sedentary desk job to a position that involves a lot of walking and they lose weight. If you have a desk job and need to lose weight, consider changing to a more active position.

Don't work night shift

By design, our bodies work best when we get plenty of restful sleep at night. Physiological processes wind down at night and then ramp back up before awakening to get us ready for the day. Working night shift makes it harder to lose weight because this works against our natural rhythm.

Don't be your own enabler

When the evening news showed firefighters cutting a large hole in the side of a house to get an 800-pound person to the hospital, the reporter asked how they got food if they couldn't get out of the house. The answer was that people brought food to them. This person had enablers contributing to their obesity. You don't want to be your own enabler. Successful weight losers will turn down people trying to sabotage their efforts.

Learn delayed fullness after a meal

Satiety is a delayed response. If I eat pizza until I'm full, I can eat 6 slices but then I'm miserable an hour later. My misery memory is easily overwhelmed by my hunger and love of pizza. If I limit my pizza intake to two slices, I feel very satisfied an hour later and not miserable. Successful weight losers will stop eating before they feel stuffed understanding fullness will come later.

Break behavior chains

If you go through the drive-thru every time you drop the kids off at soccer practice you simply must do something else to break this chain. If you eat snacks when you sit in your comfy TV chair you have to break this chain. If you overeat high calorie foods at parties, it is important to strategize against this to achieve a healthy weight. We develop many unhealthy behavior chains that become automatic. Successful weight losers form new behaviors to break these chains. Habits form with repetition over time. Once you get in the habit of a healthy behavior, it will feel automatic over time.

Plan your eats, eat your plan

Scuba instructors teach you to plan your dive and dive your plan. If you follow a shark with your video camera and stray from your dive plan, you could become separated from your dive buddy putting both lives at risk. Plan your dive and dive your plan. Successful weight loss requires planning out a calorie deficit and then eating your plan. Straying from the plan could be hazardous to your health. If someone brings a cake to work it will be very clear that this doesn't fit into your calorie plan for the day. If you know you are going to a high calorie party after work, you can minimize your calories during the day. Plan your eats. Eat your plan.

Put yourself in a position to win

So you've planned your eats and you plan to eat your plan but then your co-workers beg you to go with them after work to that cool Italian place by the mall. Every time you've gone there, you eat a large pasta entree, a Death by Chocolate dessert and down a couple glasses of cabernet sauvignon. Joining the group at 5 o'clock does not qualify for putting yourself in a position to win. Successful weight losers are steadfast about avoiding nutritional mine fields such as these and refuse them with stubborn determination.

Replacement

Stopping an unhealthy behavior leaves a noticeable void. Successful weight losers fill that void with a healthy behavior to reduce the chances of flipping back into bad habits. One of my patients, when stressed, used to eat chocolate. Now she goes for a walk to relieve stress. She gets her 10,000 steps per day and is healthier to show for it.

Repeat behaviors until they become habit

A habit forms by repeating a behavior over time. Healthy habits will not feel natural at first. They take time. Successful weight losers work through the awkward transition until the healthy habit that replaced a bad habit feels natural.

Reward yourself

Reward systems work. Your 13-year old cannot play video games until he cleans his room. Pick a favorite thing that is important to you and make a deal with yourself. I cannot buy a new pair of shoes until I lose 30 pounds. I cannot watch TV unless I stay on my eating plan and get my 10,000 steps in for the day. For weight loss, best to pick non-food rewards. And when you reach your goal weight, it's time for a very large, well-deserved reward.

Stop making excuses

A famous songwriter once said, "Waiting for inspiration is for amateurs. Professional songwriters get to work." Excuses never helped anyone lose weight and many excuses are dangerous attitudes. *I can't exercise. I hate ALL vegetables. No one is going to tell me what to do. Nothing ever works so I'm not going to even try. The nutritionist made me mad so I'm never going back.* Successful weight losers stick to their plan for eating and calorie burning regardless of outside influences and circumstances. Nothing will stand in their way to success.

Cancer patients prioritize their chemotherapy and radiation therapy appointments above everything else. You never hear them miss a cancer treatment because their ankle was sore or the receptionist was rude to them or because it was raining outside. They are fighting a disease and the fight gets first priority over everything. Obesity is a serious disease that will shorten your life. It will reduce the quality of the life you have left. The fight gets priority over everything else. Don't make excuses and skip your chemotherapy appointments. Don't make excuses and skip your intake planning and burning of calories. Highly successful weight losers put their health plan first above everything else. They don't make excuses and life-shortening diseases lose the fight.

Be open-minded

Frank Zappa once said, "*A mind is like a parachute. It doesn't work if it is not open.*" Closed minded people say things like, "Oh, I will never try that" or "That never works" or "I can't do broccoli". Unsuccessful weight losers have long lists of closed mindedness. They successfully back themselves into a corner of failure and then bring out another long list of external things to blame for no results. Successful weight losers are open-minded and their results show.

Relax

Some patients eat in reaction to negative emotions such as stress or anxiety. Learning how to better deal with stress and anxiety can be an important skill to rid phantom hunger and achieve a healthy weight. An important part of this is learning how to relax. Easy to say. Harder to do. Read books. Do yoga. Meditate. Learn how to relax. It will help your weight loss.

Fitness

If you hold a cat by the tail, you learn things that cannot be learned in any other way.

Mark Twain

Don't say the E word

If you say the word "exercise" to an obese person, an immediate image enters their mind of a ripped young trainer screaming insults at them while the rest of the gym snickers behind their hands. This is not helpful. The good news is that you don't have to join a gym and try to look like a body builder to achieve a healthy weight. I had a patient lose over 400 pounds simply by walking every day. It really doesn't have to be complicated. But you do have to burn more calories than you eat to lose weight. Many people don't realize that calorie burning will raise your metabolism for hours even after you step off the treadmill.

There are scientists who state that it's not just calories in and calories out. This is true. Our bodies don't light broccoli on fire and measure the energy it produces like a calorimeter. Lighting fat on fire certainly does give off a lot of energy. Have you ever seen a grease fire? And oftentimes patients lose weight before their burned calorie number exceeds their eaten calorie number. There are also medical conditions that make it harder to lose weight so it is much more complicated than that. But in those patients, they have to burn even MORE calories than they eat, so it really is kind of about calories in and calories out. If you tell a patient not to worry about calories, then you shouldn't worry when they're not losing weight.

Fortunately, not all personal trainers are ex-Marines with a whistle. Many excellent ones can help you achieve your weight loss goals without screaming or whistles. The key is to find one that you like. A personal trainer will reduce your chances of getting a program-ending injury. Also, buy yourself a nice pair of tennis shoes. I see way too many people dust off a pair of sneakers from the attic and end up with an injury which brings their weight loss to a screeching halt.

The key to stay motivated is to avoid injury and find a calorie burning activity that you enjoy. Focus on small steps and realistic goals. Reward yourself. Burn calories with friends, family and co-workers. Make calorie burning a social activity instead of social eating.

Burn more calories than you consume

There is only one secret to weight loss: calorie deficit. Weight *gain* is a result of caloric excess – eating more than you burn. Weight *loss* is a result of caloric deficit – burning more than you eat. Simply put, we must burn more calories than we eat to lose weight. If you are trying to lose weight and not tracking eaten calories against burned calories, it will be much harder for you to achieve success. The most powerful habit I consistently see among my most successful weight losers is calorie tracking. If you only selected one habit out of this entire book to help you lose weight, this would be the one to pick.

In the fascinating modern day age we live in where we carry a computer ("phone") around all day, there are excellent apps that make calorie tracking easy. Search "calorie tracker" in the app store. The two most popular are "My Fitness Pal and "Lose It". These are robust programs, but you have to be honest with yourself and track 100% of everything you eat or drink during the day.

Too many people try to starve themselves into a calorie deficit with no calorie burning. Or they will try to gym their way into a calorie deficit with no plan for calorie intake. Successful weight losers will combine a well thought out calorie intake plan, calorie burning plan and pay attention to the mental stuff to achieve and maintain a healthy weight.

Look for excuses to burn calories

They say lazy people make the best engineers because they find an easier way to do things. Years of brilliant inventions have drastically reduced our need to walk and move. We have radically migrated toward less and less movement. We constantly search for ways to not burn calories. With the obesity epidemic in the United States, we now need to look for ways to burn calories. We need to go back in time. There was a day when we had to walk to the meat store to get meat, walk to the dairy to get milk and then walk to the bakery to buy bread. If you really want to go back in time, there was a day when we had to chase a buffalo for hours and spear it so we could gorge on protein once a week. Now, with a click of the mouse, we can have meat, milk and bread delivered to the house. The current trend of fast food home delivery will be a disaster for the obesity epidemic.

There are thousands of ways to burn calories. The best calorie burning activity is one you will do. Look for things you enjoy such as going for a walk, Appalachian clogging, Wii Fit or whatever you will sustain. Also, mix it up to keep it interesting. Calorie burning for weight loss has two components: cardiovascular fitness and muscle toning. Cardiovascular fitness involves getting your heart rate and respiratory rate up such as brisk walk or jogging or treadmill or cycling, etc. Muscle toning is important. Muscle mass decreases as we age and become less active. This lowers our BMR – basal metabolic rate – making it harder to lose weight. The only way to reverse this is to tone your muscles. The best muscles to tone for weight loss are the big ones – the thigh and butt muscles. Step exercises (step up, step down) are great for this. Everyone has a step in their home and if you don't you can buy a cheap kitchen step. Do this while you watch television and watch the scale go down.

Successful weight losers look for any reason to burn extra calories. They park farthest from the door to force them to walk more. They buy standing desks for their office. They don't take elevators, escalators or moving sidewalks at the airport. They use the bathroom two floors up and take the stairs. These are called ADL's – Activities of Daily Living. ADL's, in a given 24-hr period, burn more calories than doing an hour on the treadmill.

Amp up your ADL calorie burning. You'll see better results in your weight loss success.

Burn calories while watching TV

Time to get creative here. You can ride an exercise bike while you watch TV. Exercise bands are great for overall toning and many of them come with an instructional DVD or online instruction. You can get these at Wal-Mart, Target, sporting goods stores or online. Take a can of beans and work your biceps while sitting on the couch in front of the TV. Go back in time. Burn more calories. Look for excuses to burn more calories.

Find fun ways to burn calories

Staying motivated is important for long-term success. Hang a calendar on the wall. Place a star or sticker on any day you meet your activity goals. You will not want to see an empty day on that calendar. Take an evening stroll with your spouse and kids. Go for walks with friends. Walk in the mall (not in the food court). Buy an energetic dog. Take a hike through a national or state park. Buy a trampoline. Buy a bike. Rock climb. Kayak. Frisbee golf. Find activities you enjoy. Successful weight losers look for sustainable solutions. The more fun it is, the more likely you are to keep doing it.

Tape the remote to the side of the TV

We need to go back to a time when we weren't the most obese nation in the world. In those days, if you wanted to change the channel on the TV, you had to stand up, walk across the room, change the channel and then walk back to the couch. Remote controls have made us gain a lot of weight. There was a time when the phone rang, you had to run into the kitchen to answer it and stand there on a short cord until the conversation was over. You also had to finger dial rotary phones. If the phone number had a lot of 9's in it, you burned a lot of calories. Today, we can sit on the couch with a snack and a high calorie sugar drink with a cell phone and a remote control and command our life like a NASA Control Center for hours without moving. Successful weight losers burn calories like we did in the 1970's when there were no remote controls or cell phones.

Walk

One of my patients lost over 400 pounds by walking. She never joined a gym. She never lifted a dumbbell. Her only calorie burning was walking. She would not go to bed until she had her 10,000 steps for the day. If she traveled with her husband, she would not let him book a hotel unless it had a treadmill.

Pedometers are cheap. Buy one. Most smart phones have a pedometer built in. iPhones have a free pedometer in the "Health" app. Your goal is 10,000 steps per day. It's OK not to start there. Buy comfortable tennis shoes, work up to 10,000 steps over time and don't injure yourself.

Many people mistakenly try to nutrition their way to weight loss with no calorie burning. Or they try to gym their way to weight loss with no regard for nutrition. And none of these things work without addressing the mental stuff. Successful weight loss is like a 3-legged stool. Take one of the 3 disciplines (mental stuff, fitness or nutrition) away and the whole thing falls down. Successful weight losers have well thought out plans for all three, they work hard, and they lose weight and maintain weight loss.

Pool exercises

One of the best-kept secrets for calorie burning is pool exercise. It is nearly 100 degrees (98.6F) inside our bodies – our core temperature. The brain defends this core temperature mightily. This is one of its high priority functions along with making the body breathe and seek food and water. Most public pools are around 78 degrees – 20 degrees below core body temperature. When you submerge an item in liquid, it quickly cools until it matches the temperature of the liquid. If you chill a bottle of wine in the refrigerator, your guests will be waiting for hours. If you submerge it in ice water, it cools much quicker. If our core body temperature dropped to 78 degrees, we would die of hypothermia. The reason our core temperature doesn't drop to match the pool temperature is that our bodies burn calories to generate heat. Pool exercises burn calories in two different ways. You burn calories with any muscle movement in the water and you burn calories to generate heat to defend your core body temperature. Pool exercises are also great for patients with joint pain because buoyancy takes weight off the joints. I see patients in wheelchairs and patients who need bilateral (both sides) knee replacement surgery because their knees are "bone on bone" – no cartilage left after carrying around extra weight for years. Telling these patients to run a 5K is unrealistic and won't work. The best solution is pool exercise.

Get a bike. Ride it every day

Some of my patients who lost over 100 pounds told me their secret was to buy a bike and ride it every day. They tell me it is easier on their sore joints and they burn more calories because the ride is more interesting and less strenuous than walking or jogging. Parents have told me they love riding as a family (everyone with helmets). Some patients have left the car in the garage and biked to work during the non-winter months.

Get a dog

When a patient tells me they just got a Labrador retriever, I tell them they are going to lose a lot of weight. I love Labradors. They have this wonderful positive attitude and zest for life. Our Lab, Bella, is so happy to see me she jumps in the air every time I walk in the door after work. When we take her for an evening stroll, she doubles our normal pace. When she sees a squirrel, we get our 10,000 steps in before the squirrel reaches the top of a tree. Dogs are wonderful companions for a happy life. A study at the University of Missouri-Columbia revealed that petting a dog can lower your blood pressure by 10%. U.S. Presidents will frequently get a dog at the White House and say it's their only friend. Do you want to increase your calorie burning and happiness? Get a dog.

Fartlek

Interval training is a great way to build muscle for weight loss.

Another term for interval training is Fartlek, which is a much funnier term. Fartlek is a Swedish term meaning, "speed play". Interval training blends continuous training for endurance and interval training for speed. An example is jogging mixed with short sprints. Add interval training to your calorie burning routine and see the results. Google "Fartlek routines". Ask your trainer to add some Fartlek to your routine.

Couch to 5k

A completely sedentary person can run a 5K after 9 weeks of training using the free Couch to 5K app. This utilizes interval training and the start-slow-and-build up method. Each session begins with a 5-minute warmup walk followed by intervals of jogging. A tone followed by a very pleasant voice will inform you when it's time to walk or jog. You end each session with a 5-minute cool down walk. You start Week 1, Day 1 with very brief intervals of jogging and lots of walking. You do this 3 days per week with rest days between. This program builds stamina and minimizes soreness and injury. Nearly everyone can do this. Successful weight losers take advantage of realistic, sustainable approaches to calorie burning instead of saying, "I'm going to run a marathon every day."

Muscle metabolism

The highest percentage of our metabolism (BMR-basal metabolic rate) comes from muscle metabolism. Muscle mass burns calories while we sleep. In a given 24-hour period, our basal metabolic rate burns more calories than we might burn running on a treadmill in the gym. The best way to boost our metabolism is to build muscle mass. This is why men tend to lose weight faster than women. Men with low testosterone (and therefore less muscle mass) will struggle to lose weight. Restoring testosterone to normal levels and building muscle with strength training can help fat burning from calorie deficit. The largest muscles in our body are the butt and thigh muscles so 10,000 steps per day builds muscle and increases metabolism.

Nutrition

"Oh, oh! I love broccoli. I make broccoli with cheese and I pick the green $#@! out – it is delicious!"

Actual quote from a patient

Calorie tracking apps

Losing weight is a battle. You need a battle plan. Army generals create a detailed plan before going into battle. Imagine the outcome if they didn't. Trying to lose weight without knowing how many calories and grams of fat and sugar you are eating is like driving to work blindfolded. Failure is in your near future if you choose the blind approach. Complex tasks require lots of information, planning and adjustment. Highly successful weight losers plan their eating for the day and then eat their plan. If you ask them how many fat grams they ate on Monday, they will probably have it memorized or open their phones and tell you within 10 seconds. They read Nutrition Facts labels in the grocery store. Every food choice is compared against their eating plan.

An extremely common scenario in every weight loss office is a frustrated patient who states, "I'm doing everything right and still not losing weight." You ask to see their calorie tracking logs and they can't produce them. They firmly state that they don't need to do tracking because they are confident they are doing everything right. You remind them to do their tracking for one week and bring it back to the office. Here, you will commonly find Gatorade (loads of sugar), handfuls of snacks throughout the day at work and at home, extra calories sneaking in here and there nearly imperceptible until you have to document 100% of your intake. Usually you find very little activity on the calorie burning side. Patients will take in 3,000 calories per day, burn less than 300 calories per day, and ask why they're not losing weight. So often patients try to nutrition their way to weight loss ignoring fitness. Others will try to gym their way to weight loss ignoring nutrition. Sometimes they do quite amazing at nutrition and fitness and ignore the mental stuff and the whole thing tumbles down – like a 3-legged stool. The market is flooded with weight loss books hyper-focused on nutrition with no mention of fitness or mental stuff. You cannot over-simplify weight loss. Successful weight loss is a complex process that fights the body's natural desire to store calories and survive.

Search "calorie tracker" or "calorie counter" in your app store. Two robust apps are "My Fitness Pal" and "Lose It". For this to work, you have to be honest with yourself and track 100% of everything you eat and drink during the 24-hour period. These apps make tracking easy. You can even scan the bar code on the package and it enters the information automatically. It saves your entries to make it easier to enter the next time if you eat the same thing. Nearly every restaurant food is in their database. Another key piece of information is the pie chart of fat/carb/protein balance. Some patients clearly favor higher carb foods and other favor fats. A balanced pie chart is an important part of eating healthy for weight loss.

Weight gain comes from caloric excess. Weight loss comes from calorie deficit. When scientists say it's not just calories in and calories out, they are correct. Some people have medical conditions that make it harder to lose weight so they require even more drastic calorie deficits so it kind of really is about caloric balance. If you tell a patient not to worry about calories, don't expect results.

Take a multi-vitamin every day

A daily multi-vitamin can help with weight loss. Calcium is needed to mobilize fat cells. Vitamin D deficiency is common since we don't spend a lot of time outdoors. Natural sunlight converts Vitamin D to its active form. Treating Vitamin D deficiency helps weight loss. B-vitamins are natural anti-depressants and help people feel more energetic.

Don't skip meals

Ravenous hunger from missing a meal can increase daily caloric intake. The drive to eat is a powerful biologic drive. The brain desperately wants you to breathe and eat. If the brain smells a hint of starvation, it panics and throws out all kinds of food seeking behavior and sends your appetite hormones through the roof. The process of weight loss fights strong compensatory mechanisms built for survival.

Some experts advocate healthy snacks between meals to control hunger. Some recommend eating 5 small meals per day. Patients benefit from these strategies through hunger control but morphing this into grazing is detrimental to weight loss success.

A common mistake is to eat nothing all day (which gets your body fully interested in preservation mode) and then eat a large dinner before going to bed (no calorie burning). This plan will leave you frustrated with poor weight loss results. A common weight loss recommendation is to eat most of your calories for breakfast and lunch while you are active during the day.

Having said this, intermittent fasting is now a popular research topic. Some early studies suggest this can improve weight loss and others suggest it may be harmful. Stay tuned for long-term study results.

Whole grains

Grains are the seeds of cereal plants such as corn, rice and wheat. Whole-grain kernels have 3 parts: bran, endosperm and germ. <u>Bran</u> is the hard outer shell, which contains fiber, minerals and antioxidants. <u>Endosperm</u> is the middle layer containing carbs. <u>Germ</u> is the inner layer with vitamins, minerals and protein. Refined grains remove the germ and bran layers leaving the endosperm. Enriched refined grains add back some of the vitamins and minerals. Whole grains have been a part of our diet since the beginning of time and are still the healthiest option. Oats are higher in fiber and protein and help lower cholesterol. Two heaping spoons of brown sugar atop oats for breakfast, however, do not count as a healthy option for weight loss.

Fiber from whole grains helps curb appetite and prevent constipation. Legumes (beans) are high in fiber and protein. Edamame (immature soybeans) uniquely contain all essential amino acids. They make great salad additions and healthy snacks.

Poop every day

It amazes me how many people think it's okay to have one BM per week. This is not okay. Patients say, "that's just me." It is not just you. That is incredibly unhealthy for your colon and that level of constipation will make you feel lousy. It is hard to lose weight when you feel lousy. You should have 1-2 BMs per day that are soft and easy to pass. If you go >24 hours without a bowel movement or your stool plops into the toilet like a stray golf ball in a pond, you are constipated. The key to a healthy GI tract is to drink plenty of water (64 ounces per day) and eat plenty of fiber. The American Heart Association recommends 25 grams of fiber per day.

A related area of active research is the "microbiome" – the balance of bacteria in our colon. Some studies suggest that the microbiome can influence weight loss. Antibiotics can kill off "good" bacteria in our colons allowing the "bad" bacteria to get the upper hand. An example of this is "C Diff" (*clostridium difficile, cdiff colitis, pseudomembranous colitis*), whereby, you develop severe watery, odorous diarrhea after taking antibiotics. This requires a specific antibiotic against *cdiff* that helps restore the colon's healthy balance of bacterial species. Probiotics are a hot topic with lots of opinions and mixed research. We don't have all the answers yet but stay tuned to these hot topics as they relate to weight loss.

Eat more fish

There is a lot to like about fish when you are trying to eat healthy and lose weight. In general, meats and beans are high protein foods. Compared to the artery-clogging saturated fats in steak, fish contains unsaturated fats and omega-3 fatty acids.

Interestingly, buffalo meat is lower in saturated fat than cow beef but fish still beats buffalo for healthier protein.

Omega-3 fatty acids in fish are essential fats. The body can make most of the types of fat that it needs except for Omega-3's. The best dietary sources of Omega-3's include fish, walnuts, flax seeds and leafy vegetables. Omega-3 fatty acids are an important part of cell membranes. They are precursors for hormones that regulate blood clotting, relaxation of arterial walls and inflammation. Omega-3 fats have been shown to help prevent heart disease and stroke. They can also improve inflammatory conditions such as lupus, eczema and rheumatoid arthritis.

The healthiest choices are baked fish. Fried fish and chips or fish served with loads of butter or high calorie sauces work hard against well-intentioned weight loss plans.

Eat slow food

Every time I have a patient in the office that has just lost over 100 pounds, I ask them what they thought the keys were to their success. Their answers over many years are the content of this book. One patient answered, "I eat slow food." I loved this answer. She explained that she used to only eat fast food and now she eats slow food. She now eats fresh, wholesome, healthy food that she prepares herself.

Work with a nutritionist

After years of chronic dieting, many patients have a lot of nutrition information, but they have no plan for calorie burning or the mental stuff that are equally critical to success. All of the highly successful weight losers I write about in this book worked with excellent nutritionists in our office. Many of these patients had a lot of misinformation or not enough information about healthy eating. Information is knowledge. Information is power. You need a lot of information and power to battle the disease of obesity. The Academy of Nutrition and Dietetics have a website, www.eatright.org, that contains a lot of useful information. You can find an expert in your area by clicking the "Find an Expert" button in the top right corner of their website. Consultation with a nutritionist can be especially valuable for vegetarians, diabetics, food allergies or patients with religious restrictions.

Don't drink calories

Liquid sugar is absorbed quickly. Your blood sugar skyrockets. Insulin levels soar. Insulin brings sugar inside the cell for storage. Your blood sugar plummets. You feel lousy. You eat more sugar to feel better. The cycle starts over and you gain weight.

Patients will come to their clinic appointment steaming mad and point their finger and shout that they are doing everything right and not losing weight. Then they take a big gulp of their fancy coffee drink containing over 1,000 calories of fat and sugar. We see this nearly every day. I see patients that lose over 30 pounds when they stop drinking high sugar sodas. In the south, its sweet tea. Many angry "perfect" patients are getting >60 grams of sugar per day from high sugar drinks. The orange coolers on the sidelines help propel the myth that sports drinks are healthy. Many patients consider fruit juices healthy. Natural sugar is stored as fat just like added sugar and high fructose corn syrup. Highly successful weight losers don't drink calories.

Alcohol in moderation

Nothing in moderation is bad for you, says the old adage. Too often, alcohol brings an otherwise well-meaning weight loss effort to a screeching halt. Highly successful weight losers have been known to have a glass of wine here and there but if it affects their weight loss, it is the first thing to go. If you feel like you can't control your drinking, get help from a professional. It could be the most important thing you ever do for your health.

Avoid high fructose corn syrup, saturated fats, trans fat, hydrogenated oils

Our movement away from fresh wholesome foods is a major contributor to the obesity crisis. The typical American diet is loaded with highly processed foods. Brilliant food chemistry created high fructose corn syrup, trans fats and hydrogenated oils.

These improve baking characteristics, shelf life and profits but do not help us maintain a healthy weight.

The food industry hydrogenates vegetable oils to change their characteristics at room temperature and improve their baking characteristics. For example, hydrogenating vegetable oils makes margarine and spreads that are solid at room temperature instead of liquid. Partial hydrogenation creates semi-solid fats that are better for baking because of the way the fat mixes with flour producing a more desirable texture in the finished product. Partially hydrogenated vegetable oils ("shortening") are cheaper than animal fats and can be tailored to a desired consistency. The finished product has a longer shelf life. The biggest problem with these is that our bodies are not good at processing them and we tend to store them as fat. Trans fats (another name for partially hydrogenated oils) have become such a major health problem, the US government requires disclosure of trans fat content on all nutrition labels. Some states and countries have banned them.

As sugar cane availability decreased, prices rose. Food chemists created a process to make food sweetener out of corn, which is plentiful and cheap in the United States. With the availability of cheap sweetener, HFCS (high fructose corn syrup) became prevalent in the American food supply. Though HFCS isn't solely to blame for the obesity epidemic, the incidence graphs of the two are quite similar. Every cell in our bodies can metabolize glucose, but only the liver can process fructose. Excess fructose is associated with fatty liver and insulin resistance that leads to type 2 diabetes.

Highly successful weight losers are knowledgeable about food additives and more likely to choose fresh, wholesome foods over brilliant food chemistry.

Learn how to read food labels

In 1990, Congress passed the NLEA – Nutrition Labeling and Education Act. This required nutrition labels on food packages that specifies nutritional contents. These help us track calories, protein, fats and carbs. Calorie tracking apps make this automatic by scanning the bar code on the package. Highly successful weight losers know how to use nutrition labels to make smart choices and their results show.

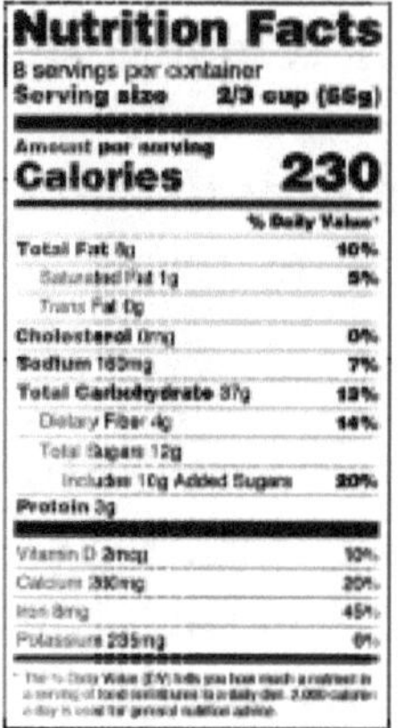

Water

70% of our body weight is water. We need about 64 ounces of water per day for healthy metabolism. Its even more important to drink plenty of water when losing weight because your kidneys work hard to eliminate metabolites from burning fat.

Patients frequently mistake thirst for hunger. If you feel hungry and its not mealtime, try drinking water. You may be thirsty. If you drink a glass of water before a meal, it may reduce caloric intake. Highly successful weight losers will typically have a bottle of water with them at all times.

Learn to enjoy fruits and vegetables

Fruits and vegetables are high in fiber, which make us feel full on fewer calories. Eating fruits and vegetables can reduce intake of higher calorie density foods. Fats are high calorie dense foods (9 calories* per gram). Carbs and proteins are less calorie dense (4 calories* per gram).

It is hard to starve yourself into a calorie deficit. Ravenous hunger is the biggest reason people stop weight loss attempts. A strategy to fight this is to eat more fruits and vegetables. They are healthy for you. Appetite studies show that fullness comes from volume of food, not caloric content. I have patients tell me,

"I hate all vegetables." This is closed mindedness and a dangerous attitude. Successful weight losers don't say this. Steamed or grilled vegetables are delicious. Try them. You will like them.

*(actual value is kilocalories which most labels abbreviate "calories")

Natural appetite reducers

Ravenous hunger brings many well-intentioned diets to a halt. Certain foods have a reputation for reducing appetite. These may help lower caloric consumption. Among them: almonds, coffee, ginger, avocado, cayenne pepper, apples, eggs, water, sweet potatoes, plums, vegetable soup, dark chocolate, tofu, wasabi, green tea and oatmeal. Healthy unsaturated fats in avocado create fullness by releasing a hormone in the duodenum call CCK (cholecystokinin). CCK is a natural appetite suppressant. Green leafy vegetables (spinach, kale) delay fat absorption in the small intestine and reduce appetite.

Normal eating

In the sixties and seventies, obesity was rare in the U.S. and we just ate – normally. By comparison, we now eat far more calories and burn far fewer calories. We need to go back in time. Distortion of our eating patterns and portion sizes is extreme. Our view of normal eating is radically different from healthy eating. We swing from out-of-control eating to highly-controlled eating and back and forth we go. We don't eat. We are either fully "ON" a diet or fully "OFF" a diet. In the middle of the road, lies a wonderfully normal eating pattern that is rational and sustainable. We used to be good at this in the 1970s.

The Mediterranean diet gets high marks for healthy eating and sustainability. Mediterranean countries have fewer deaths from coronary heart disease than the U.S. and northern Europe. Their normal diet is high in fruits, vegetables, whole grains, beans, nuts, seeds and olive oil (unsaturated "healthy" fat). They eat fish, poultry, beans and eggs weekly. They eat much less dairy and red meat compared to the U.S. They also share meals with family and friends and are more physically active. Of course, if you live in the

Mediterranean, you don't call this a weight loss diet. This is normal eating for you. The U.S. News and World Report just named the Mediterranean Diet the #1 diet for the year 2020.

Behavior repetition becomes habit over time. We need to eat normally again, until it becomes habit – like we used to.

Get the cigarettes out of the house

Not talking about smoking here. We're talking about bowls of snacks and candy sitting around the house. If you want to stop smoking, you gotta get the cigarettes out of the house. If you want to lose weight, you gotta get the bowls of snacks and candy and junk food out of the house. Self-control is better than will power. Don't let your lack of self-control put yourself in a situation that requires massive will power. Put yourself in a position to win. Get the cigarettes out of the house (and car and office and purse and...).

Liquid protein fast

There is a psychological principle called stimulus reduction. A liquid protein fast can be a great way to reduce stimuli, hit the reset button and jump start weight loss. This is like turning your computer off and then back on again. Mapping out a course from your current diet to eating healthy can be overwhelming. Too many decisions. One simple starter strategy is to go from your current diet to a liquid protein fast. For two weeks, you eat nothing but protein drinks that add up to 800 calories per day and 60 grams of protein. Commercial forms of this include Optifast and Medifast. You can DIY this with protein drinks such as Slim Fast, etc. These are called VLC diets (very low calorie) and they're best done under the supervision of a physician.

Control your environment

You still have to buy chips and cookies for your husband, the office group at work goes to a fast food joint for lunch every day and you can't miss business discussions or team building so good intentions for healthy eating are quickly tossed to the side. Highly successful weight losers control their environment. They don't let it control them. They don't buy unhealthy foods for the family. They plan and prepare a healthy lunch to avoid the inevitable high calorie meals their co-workers eat every day of the week. If their friend wants to meet for lunch on Saturday, they go for a walk instead. If it's not on the plan, they won't give in.

Traveling for business adds a challenging element to this because you don't have control of your eating options like you do at home. This requires a lot more planning and preparation to access healthy eating on the road. Highly successful weight losers will be in the hotel gym instead of watching TV in their room. They control their environment.

Mustard

Most of us don't like dry sandwiches. Mayo is a high calorie food. Mustard is a very low calorie food. Over a year's time, this simple switch can reduce serious calories. Mustard also contains turmeric, a natural antioxidant and anti-inflammatory. Mayo made with olive oil is better than regular mayo but mustard is still a healthier choice that fits easier into normal calorie eating plans.

Cook at home

Realtors tell me that many of the houses they show have spotless ovens with the owner's manual still taped inside. Microwaves, on the other hand, have multiple stains from chronic food explosions. In the skinny seventies, we gathered around the dinner table at night to enjoy a freshly prepared meal from Mom. We rarely do that anymore. We've gotta go back in time. We need to cook more meals at home where we're not subjected to highly processed foods with brilliant food chemistry. An online search for "healthy cooking" or "healthy recipes" will uncover many cookbooks, magazine, videos and websites.

Balanced diet (carbs/fats/protein)

We are pendulum swingers. We go from eating excessive carbs and then swing to highly restricted carbs and then back to overdoing carbs. We sugar crash. We swing from way too much fat to limited fat. High-fat diets make us crave high-fat foods. We swing from all-you-can-eat protein and little carbs until our body craves carbs and we swing way back. Excess carbs are stored as fat. Excess protein is stored as fat. Excess fat is stored as fat. All the while, there is this marvelous normal eating pattern that we did in the past when obesity was rare. We have to go back in time. We weren't designed to keep swinging back and forth from excess to over-control. Too often, we try to nutrition our way to weight loss, ignoring fitness or vice versa. We ignore the mental stuff. Success is a 3-legged stool.

Get your minimum protein requirements

Unless you are training for a marathon or really hitting the dumbbells in the gym, women need about 45 grams of protein per day; men need about 55 grams. The human body is very re-sourceful. If we don't eat enough protein, our bodies get it from our muscle but this lowers metabolism (BMR-basal metabolic rate). Muscle wasting can make the scale look better but you feel weaker and have a lower metabolism. Excess protein is stored as fat but not eating minimum requirements can lower metabol-ism. Proteins suppress our appetite over a longer period of time. Carbohydrates increase insulin, which stores glucose as fat, and then blood sugar lowers making you feel hungry.

Buy a Crock-Pot

Patients frequently complain that they're simply too busy to cook meals at home. Buy a Crock-Pot. The online recipes are nearly infinite. You dump stuff in it in the morning and it cooks dinner while you're at work. When you get home and open the door it smells like your mother has been slaving over the stove all day. Slow food can be really fast.

Don't eat after 7:00PM

Studies suggest that weight loss is more successful when you eat your calories in the morning and not in the evening. This can be tough because many patients describe boredom hunger in the evening but highly successful weight losers strategize and plan for this.

Portion distortion

If you talk about pasta portion size, the image of a huge steaming bowl of spaghetti and meatballs from our favorite Italian place immediately pops into my mind. The problem is this should feed four people. Not one. But I eat all of it. No doggie bag necessary, thank you. That was delicious as usual. 20% tip.

If restaurants served normal portions, no one would go there. Our ideal of normal portions has become so distorted, it is hard to bring us back to reality in terms of how little food we actually need to sustain life. And it doesn't help that most lunch places have a cookie the size of my head sitting next to the cash register. Nowadays, when we say we ate one cookie, we're talking about the caloric equivalent to a sleeve of Oreos. We've got to go back in time. We've got to re-establish normal portions. We've got to use smaller plates, eat slow, chew more, eat higher calorie dense foods first for fullness, realize fullness is delayed and only eat in the dining room.

Understand the insanity of eating fried potatoes three times per day

The serving size for fried potatoes in a healthy diet is zero. The problem is that we're consciously eating them three times per day. Everyone knows that you get the hash brown oval in the morning, waffle or curly fries for lunch and then steak fries for dinner and they taste much better with high fructose corn syrup ketchup. This "norm" has been a disaster for the American diet. Norms like this are literally killing us. Highly successful weight losers skip the fries. Anyone interested in losing weight should do the same.

Meal prep on Sunday

People that work full-time and rely on nearby restaurants for lunch struggle with weight loss. Highly successful weight losers control their environment. They brown bag it. They meal prep on Sundays and place portions in freezer containers for the rest of the week.

Wean off dessert

Giant deserts in restaurants have become too much of a norm. To lose weight, we need to wean ourselves off giant desserts. Fruit is a better way to wean yourself from the unhealthy habit of a sugary dessert. Fruit smoothies made at home are healthier than sweets made from highly processed materials and HFCS.

Nothing in moderation is bad for you. Having cake on your birthday is normal. If you're trying to lose weight and it's not your birthday, cake would be a terrible choice. It is a high sugar, high fat, high calorie food. Eating sweets skyrockets your blood sugar which increases insulin levels which takes all that blood sugar and converts it into fat. This lowers your blood sugar, which makes you ravenously hungry two hours later. Sweets can ruin weight loss efforts.

Learn how to eat healthy in restaurants

Avoiding restaurants is easy to say and difficult to do. I would have a hard time avoiding all restaurants. Many of my patients travel and entertain for work. Taking clients to restaurants for business meetings is an important part of their occupation. More and more, restaurants offer healthier selections, smaller portions, baked chicken and fish with no high calorie sauces. You can order salad dressing on the side. Some of my business travelers struggle to lose weight. Others knock it out of the park. Highly successful weight losers find a way to eat smaller and healthier portions in restaurants and entertain while sipping on tonic water and lime instead of a high calorie cocktail.

Stay current

Weight loss is a rapidly changing field with much research. Given the complexity of the human body and its strong desire for survival, it is unlikely that we will have a magic pill in our lifetime. Obesity is a complex disease. The only way to go wrong is to oversimplify it. The solution for successful weight loss is complex and requires a lot of work. It is a curable disease but the cure doesn't come easy.

Do it

Seriously. Put down this book and go do it. Make changes today. Look for any excuse to reduce eaten calories. Look for any excuse to burn extra calories. Make small but meaningful changes. Set realistic goals that are sustainable without injury. Yes, it takes hard work, but this isn't cancer. Obesity is a curable disease. Godspeed.

Never give up!

A common mistake while trying to achieve a healthy weight is to give up too early. Many people do everything right but they don't see a big change on the scale so they give up. If you're doing everything right, keep plowing through. Persistence pays. The scale will catch up with you. You will see success. You will be glad you stayed in the game.